CELEBRATING PREGNANCY

Again

Restoring the lost joys of pregnancy
after the loss of a child

by Franchesca Cox

DEDICATION

Dedicated to my 'rainbow' babies, Joseph Alexander and Evelyn Jane. The beautiful gifts who restored more hope and love into my world than they will ever know.

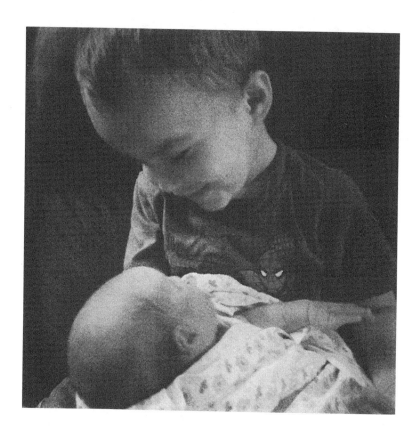

TABLE OF CONTENTS

Chapter 1

THE DAY THAT CHANGED EVERYTHING

I can remember the twenty week ultrasound like it was yesterday. I was a first time mama, buried deep in a fog of bliss, not quite grasping the sheer miracle growing inside me at the time.

Was I happy? Oh, yes. Our short marriage had a rocky start and sad to say, the problems we were working through were still present while I carried our first child. Of course, everyone has problems, but I wish - if given the chance - that I could go back in time and whisper a few things to my younger, pregnant self. No problem is worth the stress, especially during pregnancy.

I don't remember the ultrasound technician's face. But I do recall the silence in the room, and how long the ultrasound was taking. Deep down inside, I had a nagging feeling that something wasn't right. Intuition perhaps? This was new. I shoved it as far out of my mind as possible because the thought was daunting and seemed unrealistic. The nagging feeling didn't last long. There was no history of anything like birth defects or miscarriage - on either side of the family. It's one of those things you subconsciously tell yourself happens to other people, not realizing that is arrogance in its purest form.

I didn't understand most of what I saw on the monitor as the technician pushed the wand over my small but growing belly. One thing I did recognize was my baby's head, which seemed large in proportion to the rest of her body. I attempted to break the silence by making a lighthearted comment about it, fully expecting the technician to brush off my hidden concern as something that 'is totally normal at this stage'.

Well, she didn't. My nagging feeling began to grow into a possibility that maybe something was really wrong, and my mommy-intuition really had nudged me for the first time. She was lost in concentration - measuring, measuring and measuring some more. She left the room with no explanation, yet no real reason to get worked up either.

Maybe this was normal - what did I know?

What should have been a twenty-five minute ultrasound and gender-finding appointment quickly turned into one of the worst days of my life. When the technician left the room, it wasn't long before my OB stepped in to take her own measurements. She scanned me, for not quite as long and told my mom and mother-in-law, who had joined us for the exciting 20-week gender finding appointment, that we would be doing the exam now, and asked them to step out. They left the room, and what she told us next changed our lives forever. There was no exam. She simply asked us to go to her to her office where she would meet us in a few minutes.

My stomach was in knots. I knew in my heart that 'normal' patients did not have to visit her office at their twenty week ultrasounds. I felt like I had one of those out-of-body experiences as I entered that clean office of hers. Movie scenes of doctors delivering terrible news to loved ones flashed through my head. This must be what it felt like in real life. Helpless. Gut-wrenching. Far from real. There was no instrumental music in the background for dramatic effect, just the hum of every day life for the clinic. Muffled sounds leaked under the door through the hallway. Life was carrying on like normal for the families in the rooms around to us, while ours was on the brink of disaster. Nurses were tied up in their day to day routines - and *this* is what it felt like to be the one to anxiously await the miracle of good or even ordinary news but understand there would be no reason to deliver such a report in privacy.

The night before Pete and I had had a feud over something I can't remember now. He ended up deciding he would be going to work instead of joining me at the ultrasound the next morning. I was upset but I knew I would never be able to change his mind. Before you start throwing rocks at him, I probably said things I shouldn't have. We were both young, immature and this was a crude wake up call to reality. Things that mattered. When the next morning rolled around, I was surprised to see him getting ready to join me instead of throwing on his navy blue uniform shirt for work. In this moment, this surreal moment of walking into the doctor's personal office, I was never more glad we were over the petty feud last night. This jolted us into adulthood like nothing else had.

Sculptures that celebrated motherhood danced along her window pane. She had paintings, too. I could see this woman loved her job, but her bedside manner was something to be desired. When she finally joined us in her office, she wasted no time getting right down to it, sans apologies or empathy. Her distinguished Spanish accent crescendoed over the bad news like a thunderstorm. She told us our baby was measuring two weeks behind, and mentioned she had seen things on the ultrasound that had given her reason to believe our baby might have a genetic disorder - some possibilities being incompatible with life. Hearing the words *incompatible with life* felt like a punch in the face. When I think of the word *compatible* I think of my version of Windows being compatible with your software program. How did my daughter suddenly become a program? I would learn later that doctors dealing with cases similar to mine throw those words around quite a bit - not for cruelty - but for frankness and honesty. As she delivered such awful news her demeanor remained stoic and lacked compassion. I wondered if our baby - this terrible reality - made her uncomfortable and maybe this was her way of dealing with such grief. She was honest and told us she was unable to give us any solid information other than what she was able to pick up on the monitor. We were referred to a high risk clinic that afternoon, that could provide us with concrete facts, a direction, maybe even a diagnosis.

My world was shaken to the core that day, but what I didn't realize right away is that pregnancy - this one and any others to follow - would never be the same. At the time I was merely trying to survive this new normal and this potential threat to my baby that I could do absolutely nothing about. Among many other things, this new reality sent ripple effects that would affect any future pregnancies. What I once took for granted - trust in my own body to deliver a healthy child - I would have to relearn, and balance meticulously with grief and guilt. Pregnancy would be redefined by this experience in many ways, but it would also present me with the challenge to seize the opportunity and my days with child that much more because I knew how very fragile life was first hand.

After the perinatologist not only confirmed our daughter's restricted growth, but also found even more symptoms for a chromosomal disorder, any hope I had was destroyed and my innocence regarding pregnancy was gone forever. We were able to save the pregnancy for nine more weeks, the last two in hospital bed rest. Jenna was born at twenty-nine weeks on May 5, 2009 and left our world much too soon after thirteen days in the Neonatal Intensive Care Unit. If I ever doubted myself and my ability to bring a healthy child into the world, I did now. Even though we were told there was nothing more than could have been done, and that this was most likely a spontaneous alignment of chromosomes and genetics, I left the hospital with empty arms and heart full of guilt. As her mother, a part of me will always feel like I failed.

Chapter 2

SUBSEQUENT PREGNANCY:
OH, THE GUILT

Thoughts on trying again were inevitable. The urge to hold my own child seemed endless, forceful and growing with strength everyday my arms were empty. The chances of having this happen again to us - what still felt like this blanket of possibilities - was fifty-fifty. My doctor was fairly certain our daughter had a chromosomal disorder that was never diagnosed. All the blood work they did for her in the NICU came back inconclusive. She had symptoms, many of them in line with Trisomy 18. Our doctor warned us if that was the case, there was a fifty-fifty chance it could happen again.

The risk was daunting, but never enough to think about *not* trying again for us. Looking back I don't know what we would have done if it had. It, no doubt, would have been the end of me.

After we lost our first child my arms literally ached to be a mommy to a living child. Of course, I missed my daughter beyond words, but I longed to be a mommy again, feel new life growing inside, and hold my own child. I had empty-arm syndrome and it was every bit emotional pain, as it was physical.

We waited for the doctor's OK and began trying again almost immediately. Not too long after trying again, I found myself staring down at the second pregnancy test I had taken in the past twelve hours. The one I took only hours before told me I wasn't pregnant but I knew something was different. I slept that night and drove to CVS Pharmacy the next morning to give a digital pregnancy test a shot. After staring at the little annoying hour glass for what felt like hours the word "Pregnant" settled over the screen.

I remember brushing with guilt for first time as joy and fear gripped my heart simultaneously on this new journey.

This is where I wish I could tell you it ended, but it didn't. It *hasn't*. As I write this book, I am almost 19 weeks pregnant with our second rainbow child.[1] Guilt is sneaky. It's not quite as bold as it was the first go-around. I know better than to cave in and let it completely ruin my day most of the time. I've learned that I deserve happiness. You do too.

---

[1] rainbow child refers to a child born after experiencing child loss

Happiness never, ever means you don't love the child you lost. It only means you are taking a small step in healing. That, is a beautiful gift. Healing is learning a new love language for the child you lost. When you first lost your child, if you were anything like me you loved your child through tears, planning special events on birthdays and anniversaries, taking pictures of their garden, taking special note of the butterflies that happened to dance by you, or maybe even through writing. But now you are in a different place. It is okay to love your lost child through celebration and happiness. It doesn't mean that you won't cry or can't do any of those things anymore, but it is time to welcome some level of joy and happiness in your heart as well. It is important to make room for it, while giving grief it's rightful place in your heart. It is the best thing you can do for your baby on the way.

When you push the guilt out (even if only for a moment at first) and let that happiness of this new life sink in, the joy of motherhood is even more precious, even more sacred than before. It is a downright miracle. I was constantly amazed at my growing belly with my son. And even more amazed that I could grow a healthy baby after my body so horribly let me down the previous year with our daughter.

You might be feeling guilty for feeling happy, wanting to decorate for the new nursery, register for baby things, or letting your friends and family throw you a baby shower. You are not alone in this. Anyone that has lost a child, if they are honest, can tell you everything baby-related afterwards tends to be bittersweet. Everyone is affected differently, so be sure to let yourself feel whatever you might be feeling at the moment. For me, that hasn't changed a bit. Pregnancy is definitely not the same, but neither are newborn clothes, infant swings, baby showers, birth announcements - the list goes on. Sometimes I see these things and a flood of memories washes over me. Even though I now have a purpose for these things, I remember what it felt like to have some of these things and suddenly not need them.

With this pregnancy I have a mantra, and I believe it is a great starting tool in controlling your mind and where you let your thoughts wander - for the sake of the baby but also for you. It is easy to let grief sweep over you, and literally steal precious moments that you can never get back. This time with your baby is sacred, and incredibly short-lived. Writing your own mantra can help you become more vigilant about intentionally celebrating this time in your life, and suppressing the fears and guilt.

"I deserve this. It is okay to dream. It is okay to hope. Pregnancy can and will be beautiful - for as many days as that may be."

Create your mantra or steal mine. Write it down. Scream it to the birds. Grab some red lip stick and paint it across your mirror. If you don't want to make such a fuss, write it on an index card and put it where you can read it everyday. You might even give yourself reminders on your phone that encourage you to stay positive.

Pregnancy feels like it lasts forever at times, but the truth is it is one of the shortest windows of your life. A window you'll never forget, so spend it right... and do what you can to celebrate this pregnancy.

The guilt had a way of keeping an uncomfortable but seemingly impossible distance from me and my son (on the way) those first few months of pregnancy. If you want to know the recipe for making a mother feel like an ultimate failure, try mixing a mother who doesn't quite know how to fit grief in her life anymore, how to adequately express her incredible love for the new child on the way, and a giant dose of guilt that is pushing and pulling her in opposite directions daily. It seems like either way you go, grieving the baby you lost, or celebrating the new baby on the way - you can't win for losing. It feels like betrayal either way.

I kept thinking, *Dear God. I wasn't built to do this. Live this. Survive this. Much less do it right.* On top of the guilt I had the surfacing fear that I was not being the mother I should be to my son.

I felt incredibly out of touch for most of the first and second trimester with my son. Toward the end of the second trimester, the movements and kicks are so forceful, so present, it is honestly impossible not to swoon over this new little person growing inside. I gave into love toward the end, but the distance has been something that always bothered me about my pregnancy with him. I maintained the distance without really trying. It became a survival mechanism.

I was afraid. I was afraid of bonding, falling madly in love all over again, and losing what I knew I could not live without.

Chapter 3

BALANCING GRIEF IN PREGNANCY

The first perinatal appointment with our son was a surreal moment. I felt pregnant, but I felt extreme loss. If I was honest I would tell you I felt disconnected from this new baby, and wanted so desperately to know the remedy to be able to fall in love easily again, love unguarded and somehow be okay with the way things had played out only months before. I missed the baby I lost, and I wanted to love this new baby for whoever he or she would become. The battle in my heart was fierce. My heart must have been telling on me. The staff still recognized me, and no doubt felt some of the bittersweetness of it all. I'll never forget a conversation that took place with my nurse Teresa during that first appointment.

"I'm worried about you." she said over her charts, then looking straight up at me. Her dark brown eyes were honest, caring but firm.

I wasn't expecting this. By this time the rest of the world had more or less forgotten about the awfulness of our daughter's passing. It was like it never happened and I was so used to being pushed in the 'get over it, and move on' direction, that it was shocking to hear someone - a professional - validate the enormity of our loss, and the ripple effects it was sending through our world. I pretended not to know what she was talking about and gave a weak, silent nod. I feared accepting that finally someone realized I was not over Jenna's death (and never would be), and being mistaken.

"I've seen others in your situation before, and your grief *will* affect this new baby if you let it." I think she might have even suggested something about counseling or anti-depressants.

Her face grew serious with her last statement. She knew how nearly impossible the next eight months would be on me. Honestly, her words scared me to pieces. *What if I couldn't do this?*

I made a pact with myself right there and then, that I would put my grief on hold - as much as humanly possible - until the baby was born. I only had eight or so more months to make sure he got here safely; and the ugly reality is I would have the rest of my life to grieve my daughter. It instantly felt like betrayal, but it might have felt even worse if I hadn't given this new pregnancy my all.

I ended up taking my nurse up on her advice and backed away from a few things for the next few months. One was the baby loss blogs I had found so much healing in reading. I still read, but not nearly as much. I began a new blog, just for my son. It was healing and helpful to me to give him his own space.

Another thing was visiting the cemetery. I can remember feeling ripped apart with guilt stepping out of the car and onto the pavement to visit my daughter's resting place as this new life grew inside. It once again felt like betrayal, like so many things did those days. There's no easy way to do this, you just learn to tread carefully. Be gentle on yourself.

I found myself going less and less. I found myself talking to her through tears at the gravesite. I would tell her about this amazing little person that would soon be joining our family, but how I wished she could have been here, too.

Every week or so I would drive into town and run around to thrift shops, Starbucks and other errands with my mother-in-law. She was one of the few people who spoke their mind, but gave me the space I needed at the same time. Her bluntness was almost comforting. I was tired of being treated like a glass vase or like losing a baby was a disease you could catch. I was extremely fragile on the inside, but I needed some sense of normalcy, and her company provided just that.

In our visits together she would try to coax me into thinking about buying baby things. Buying anything *baby* was not even an option for me with my first rainbow pregnancy. It was too devastating to even think of piling more baby crap to our already large baby collection that I felt like we might not ever use. After a while, it not only stings to look at, it feels like it is mocking you. I wasn't about to put myself, my faith, my heart, my hopes out there like that. She read this as *not being excited about the new baby.* I can see that. Maybe in truth, I wasn't.

I know and knew then that happy endings were not a guarantee. I was skeptical about miracles. I prayed for this baby, sure. But out of sheer desperation. Excitement wasn't really the word for it. I was driven by fear that he would come early and we would end up riding that horrible NICU roller coaster only to end with another devastating aftermath of crushed dreams.

The world around you might not understand why you aren't just giddy over this new pregnancy, or jumping up and down (okay, maybe not literally) about getting the chance to buy baby things, and decorate a nursery. The world around you may read this, as they did with me, as not really wanting this new baby or being excited. This can only increase the guilt you already might be feeling. The pressure from others definitely had me feeling even more guilt that I was already feeling. Becoming pregnant again already felt like betrayal for some reason, and then not giving this baby the excitement that I knew he or she deserved - it was an upward battle.

With the first rainbow pregnancy I was pretty firm and laid down the foundation pretty early for friends and family with what I could handle and what I was just not able to do. Some liked it, some probably hated it but most were completely fine with my decisions. You are the one that has to sleep at night with your choices, and if it gives you peace buying and planning for this new baby then do it! There is no right or wrong here. It is all just survival from here until the baby's arrival. Will it get easier? It is very likely, that the closer you get to your baby's due date, and maybe even feeling them kick around, things might start to lighten up for you, but even if they don't, the most important thing right now is your well-being which in turn means baby's well-being: do what is right for you.

Another milestone was planning for the baby shower. Or I should say baby shower *talk*. That was something else I dreaded. First of all, the crowd. No one sitting in that crowd would be able to understand why opening a Noah's ark gift bag filled with fluffy baby blankets would suddenly and without warning send me into a blubbering mess. I did not want to mask how I was handling this pregnancy by putting on a face, or apologize for it either. After all, no one sitting in that room truly understood just how bittersweet and messed up this whole thing was.

So we waited. My well-meaning friends and family were skeptical about waiting on the baby shower until after the baby came, but they ultimately let me have my way. And can I just say, it was perfect. I got to open gifts with my beautiful baby boy cuddled safely in my arms.

I am not advocating against having a baby shower before the baby's arrival, but I am wanting to get across a point - you should be in control, because only you know what you can handle. Be cautious of letting your well-meaning friends and family pushing you in a direction you are uncomfortable with. I have talked to dozens of baby loss mothers who were able to handle the traditional baby shower, before baby was born. I think they are rockstars for it, too. But personally I knew that was more than I could handle, and I was okay at the end of the day with my choice.

Chapter 4

TRUSTING AGAIN

I'll be the first to admit that I was *not* (read am not) the *prime* example of what a Christian who loves Jesus should do, say, think or act like after losing a baby. At first, I think it was shock that prevented me from a lot of things, one being losing my mind.

I was cocooned in this shock-bubble for a long time, months perhaps. As the bubble began to thin out, and finally pop -- reality began to set in and I became not just disappointed in my own body for ultimate failure, but devastated that God did not come through like I had prayed so hard he would. I've heard a few Christians thank him years down the road for the journey, the way things turned out, the lessons, etc, etc., etc. I applaud them, but I am not one of them. I see no purpose worth the loss of a child, but I have found meaning in the loss. I am thankful for the gifts along the way that I have gained since her loss. But I am selfish and would trade them all *in a heartbeat* to hold her beautiful, tiny body again. I'd trade it all for a normal pregnancy, for a normal life and for ignorance.

That being said, my faith has been shaken to the core. What once was black and white suddenly became this messy canvas with splatters of paint and dirt menacing the clean white surface. There were gashes torn, rending permanent scars throughout, without rhyme or reason. The canvas was devastating to look at. The canvas I once admired so deeply. The snow white canvas that used to make sense. The faith I no longer recognized. Where do you go from utter disappointment? When, literally, the world no longer makes sense?

It seemed out of the good grace of God my faith did get me through those first few days and weeks following my daughter's death. I felt Heaven, unspeakable peace and, call me creepy, but I even felt my daughter - so close those first few days and weeks of mourning. My faith in God had gotten me through her *death*. But my faith soon after began to suffer as the permanence of this scar settled deep in my bones and grief began to do her work. The pain was penetrating, lasting, never-ending. I had never known a love so great; a loss so deep.

While her death nearly killed me, the aftermath made me long for death even more. The days, weeks and months of dwindling phone calls and visits. Spoiled flowers and crumpled flower petals on the hard wood floors. Cards once written with tear stains whose voices now rarely spoke of my loss, our daughter. The faith I once clung to for all of life's past (and now trivial) problems, no longer seemed capable of carrying the weight of this aftermath.

This faith that was bruised throughout seemed completely incompetent to carry me through another possible pending disaster. Another beautiful life. Another nine or so months of waiting.

Black and white was gone forever, and so was my premature notion of faith.

The most obvious result of this devastation was my loss of trust in God. My train of thought was not the most admirable, but it was rational. Of course, ration and reason are hardly ever in sync with the mind of God.

If he could have saved her - and he could have - and chose not to, how do you put your faith in a God like this?

I know, right? I'm horrible. But that is where my mind constantly went throughout my first pregnancy after loss. The *how?*

I can honestly say I trusted that God could keep our son safe, and that he would, but it was out of pure desperation. Not love. My faith was no longer fueled with passion for the love I once felt toward God. I wish I could travel back into time and redo that entire pregnancy. I was torn between grief and precious new life, and my faith was stretched endlessly. It was all about survival, and it seemed that if God could just decide to take my child, I had better just put my trust in him. My mindset was full of misconceptions of the love of God. There is honestly so much I don't remember from that pregnancy, and I have to chalk it up to so much fear being present.

I wish there was a cure. A magic formula. A one-two-three, repeat after me, and you'll be fine- remedy. But there isn't.

I am not going to lie and say it's easy to throw both hands in the air, and put your heart and hopes on the line - again - when you know all too well how it ended the last time you tried. It is painstaking. Excruciating. It makes absolutely no sense at times. But... you must be willing to cure your mindset of God first. You must be able to see God as love in order to truly believe he is on your side. That he is fighting for you, and your baby every step of the way. He really is.

I will tell you that as time has passed and I am now on my second subsequent pregnancy my heart is almost thankful for the waiting that comes with pregnancy. It is trying. It is *extremely* trying. It is borderline impossible. Especially those long periods between ultrasound appointments, or hearing that precious heartbeat, or feeling those amazing little kicks. But, the waiting? It is almost like a reminder now. A reminder to cherish each moment with this new baby. Because we all know it could be our last moment, we have the privilege (yes, privilege!) of treating each moment with special care and appreciation - like none other.

Think of it as a dare. A dare to embrace the moment. The next five minutes if that is all you can do. Instead of allowing fear to grip your heart, cast it down - even if for just a moment - and let that love pour in. In I John, God says, "perfect love casts out fear".

"There is no fear in love; but perfect love casteth out fear: because fear hath torment. He that feareth is not made perfect in love." - I John 4:18

Relish in the beauty of this pregnancy. The sheer miracle of life growing inside you. It is an impeccable privilege. When you allow that love to take over, and welcome this face of God, even in the aftermath of your grief, a sense of healing takes place. You get to know the love of God on a much more intimate level. That trust is being restored. And steps toward real healing is taking place.

Sometimes I think when my husband sees me smiling down at my belly, he can't help but wonder what it feels like. He's even asked in the most curious, wonderstruck voice, "What does it *feel* like when they kick?"

"Like magic." I'll usually tell him without hesitation. And in that moment I feel so humbled (and a little bad for him), to be chosen as the one to carry new life into this little family of ours.

Chapter 5

THE WORLD AROUND YOU

It had only been a few months since our loss when it suddenly felt like our world was imploding. It was not just our loss we were dealing with, but the expectations of those around us and the assumption that we were not only past our grief, but ready to handle everyone else's issues. Pete was my rock. He never let things penetrate. I, on the other hand, felt completely wiped out by grief and extremely vulnerable, trying not to lose my sanity as this new pregnancy progressed.

The problems that used to seem so big and so heavy now seemed minuscule and insignificant. You get tunnel vision with grief, and rightfully so. Especially when you have just buried your own child. When you hear others complain about their transmission going out, their finance issues, their marriage problems, or my personal favorite - their children - it all gets a little frustrating. It did for me.

Instead of wrapping up gifts or baking cupcakes to revel this new baby's arrival, it was more of a 'I'm having another baby, so *please* back off' announcement. Have I already told you I wish I could go back and do some things? Because that would have been one of them. The pressures of others around me - not only rushing me in my grief over my daughter - but unloading with their own problems, and now with this new baby was just enough to make me lose it.

The announcement wasn't anything special or planned. Mostly because I was afraid of how this pregnancy might end, instead of leaning into hope.

When we realized that this baby was not only growing, but even a little big for his age, I would be lying if I didn't tell you that a little hope did finally come into the picture. I gained a little more confidence in my ability to bring a healthy child into this world. The good news reports from each doctor's appointment were like music to my ears. But even so, the weeks between appointments felt like years. I knew how many things could go wrong in such a short amount of time. I knew that *nothing* is guaranteed, which is why it always frustrated me beyond measure when others would try to reassure me, and silence my fears by saying "Everything is going to be okay."

No one can possibly know that. No one.

Almost every time I heard those words I took a deep breath and held my tongue, because anything I had to say would come out sounding like I just wanted to rehash what our little family had been through or worse - trying to obligate others into joining my pity party. Of course, seeking out sympathy had nothing to do with it. What they could not understand was that losing our firstborn severed my happy-go-lucky fantasy about pregnancy forever. My innocence was gone and the possibility of losing this baby too was a looming nightmare.

It is very likely that how ever you choose the share the good news, the world around you will let out a huge sigh of relief. The common misconception is that this new baby will not only solve all your problems caused by your loss, but also bring back the person you used to be. The person you were before you suffered the loss of a child. Nothing could be farther than the truth.

I must have been only about sixteen weeks along with my son or so, when someone made a remark that had me scratching my head. I was too stunned to reflect how I truly felt.

"Aren't you so happy your oldest will be a boy?" she smiled like it was the biggest blessing in the world. And it was, and it wasn't. "I was so glad when we found out we would have a boy as the oldest."

I nodded silently. Just stunned. There was so much I wanted to say, but it seemed infinitely pointless.

Did she completely forget that Jenna was still, and would always be our first? That in some alternate reality, I would have a *girl* as my oldest, and nothing could be more perfect *than that?*

I know in my heart of hearts the comment was made without much thought, and most definitely not intended to wound. There were many times I had comments like this come my way, implying that Joseph was our first, as if Jenna never existed. There is almost nothing more painful that feeling like the child you lost has been forgotten.

Since we had lost our only child, and I was carrying new life the most common question from strangers was "Is this your first?" That question always made me wonder if they really wanted to know the truth.

I was usually pretty bold and answered gently, but honestly. Two things would happen at this point. Their eyes would get big, completely mortified by the what I just told them or they would give me their sentiments and walk away as quickly as possible. Occasionally, they wouldn't walk away, but open up with their own story of loss, or that of a friend or family member.

This land of pregnancy after loss makes me think of a war zone. No matter what side you are on, both sides are vulnerable. The land mines are in the most unsuspecting places. Treading this land carefully can be exhausting for both parties. The best thing you can do for your baby on the way, is to not dwell on the comments that sometimes feel loaded and hurtful. In the end, it just isn't worth the stress it might bring on you and baby.

It is amazing to me that through our loss, and the two subsequent pregnancies how jarred I felt, like it was a different planet altogether. And mostly, it has stayed the same if you really think about it. *I* am the one that has changed. Drastically. I have had many friends fall away, and new friends come to my side. More than anything I have been completely surprised by *who* has stayed, and who has moved on. Grief has a way of separating and bonding like almost nothing else. And grief has gifted me with some of the most unexpected friendships.

The best thing you can do for yourself and this beautiful new life growing inside, is to keep a smile in your heart. Surround yourself - as much as possible - with people who give you your space, understand on some level that this new pregnancy is anything but easy, and who love you regardless of who you have become since your loss.

It is likely that well-meaning people will assume that this new baby should be making everything better. Almost treating this new baby like you found a missing piece to your puzzle. Of course, the piece that is missing is forever gone, and you are learning to live without it.

My biggest mistake was bottling up, instead of being open with family and friends - people that I assumed should have known better. There were times it was probably best that I didn't say anything because nothing would have changed. There were times, however, that I should have spoken up. I gave people who had never lost a child *too much credit.* I don't say that to be ugly. It's just the truth. They didn't and they don't know any better. What rocked my world forever, rocked their lives for about 36 hours before they were able to flip on the television and enjoy a good episode of Friends. Of course, they didn't fully understand the enormous way our daughter's death was still affecting us. It blew my mind. My heart shattered into tiny smithereens every time someone else suggested that Joseph was our first, or that this new child was going to somehow 'fix' our grief.

The truth is he would bring more healing in his birth to our hearts than we could even imagine, but he would never be able to replace our daughter, or erase our loss. He would never be expected to. There was still, and there would always be that void that only our first child was meant to fill.

Don't do what I did. Save your heart. Speak up. Let others know that you are very much grieving, and very much wanting this new child. Let them know having such strong, conflicting emotions in one single heart is enough to make you explode. Let them know the new baby is loved beyond words, but he/ she will never replace the one you lost. Let them know it's okay that they don't always know what to say, or how to say it. Let them know that allowing you to be honest with them is invaluable. Above all let them know how you feel. It might or might not sound like what I just said, but in the end honesty will save a lot of friendships and at the same time, it might cost you some. But in the end, what is friendship without transparency?

Something that really kicked my faith in the shins was being told by fellow Christians that I should not be grieving since our daughter was in Heaven, and no longer in pain. This advice was all coming during my pregnancy with my son, which happened to be only months after our loss. This advice was also coming from people I once held on a metaphoric pedestal. I trusted them. But inside I was crushed. You really can't help how you feel. And it is impossible to harness grief, let alone grief with all the raging pregnancy hormones. I quickly became frustrated with religion, church and even God. Again, this became something I kept to myself - not wanting to create a mess where we certainly didn't need one. The only practical solution felt like keeping these people at arms length, right along with God since it seemed like they knew exactly what he said about my grief and how I should be handling things.

Can I just say this was not the ideal solution? My image of God became marred. It became harder and harder to love a God that seemed only capable of judging me while my heart was completely broken.

If you are being faced with a similar situation, I beg you - I really do - to seek the face of God for yourself. Don't let other well-meaning Christians taint who God really is for you. First, you must understand they are not in your shoes. They have absolutely no idea (even though they might act like they do) how they might handle your loss, your pregnancy and all the things that seem to be thrown at you during this time. Second, the promise of Heaven does not fix everything. It just doesn't. Not on this side. It will one day, but as we live and breathe today, Heaven is our infinite comfort in loss, not the solution to our broken hearts.

For some reason, even though I was pregnant again I still felt jarred around other expecting mothers. It might have been the loss of innocence. It might have even been the vibe I received from them. I suppose I can't blame them. If I was in their shoes, I wouldn't know how to act around me either.

For me, the pregnancy symptoms - the sickness, backaches, weight gain, swelling, etc... it just didn't matter.

A gift for you

Liz – I hope this book helps you or at least gives you some comfort, like it did for me <3 Aja

I was not interested in swapping pregnancy pet peeves. Other expecting mamas couldn't understand why I would say things like "I just want hear him cry."

Maybe it's because the cry wasn't the most remarkable thing about being a mom to them. But it would be to me - at first. It would mean life. It would mean he could breathe on his own without medical intervention. We never heard Jenna cry. All I remember after the emergency c-section with her is a quiet room. Feet scurrying. My husband trying to follow what was happening as they rushed this tiny baby right out of me into the arms of the neonatology team on hand. I learned later she stopped breathing at birth. She was resuscitated.

I got weird looks when those words slipped out. But they were yearnings from the heart. I so longed to relate to someone who had walked this road of pregnancy after loss before. Thankfully, I did find a community. Unorthodox to my real life family and friends, I found women from all over the world who had been through what I had been through, or similar online.

I remember reading Carly Marie's Water Babe blog, for her last beautiful daughter. All her reflections made so much sense to me.

Some of my other blog friends began getting pregnant, or were already pregnant after their losses, and it was reassuring and somewhat satisfying to read that someone else felt these conflicting emotions.

Finding this community was invaluable, even if it was through a computer screen. Part of community is being okay with where you are at, what you are feeling and who you might be becoming. Being able to read something and have that 'ah-ha!' moment, or cry "YES! Me too!" over a computer screen, while your husband glances back at you in the middle of watching a football game to make sure you're okay.

Community was pivotal to my healing, and it will be to yours. Even if your community is one person, a local support group, an online forum, or a blog community - my hope and prayer is that you will find the person(s) you need to get through this time in your life. The people that will make you feel less crazy, and encourage you when the rest of the world is pushing you to be a normal, excited expecting mother.

At about twelve weeks pregnant with my son, one of my worst fears came true with I began spotting one afternoon. I felt incredible guilt, as if I caused this to happen. Pete caught me crying in the bathroom, and I just kept repeating "it's not my fault, I didn't do this..." He kept shaking his head, not quite understanding why I even thought he was assuming it was my fault at all. But inside I was the one that felt responsible. I honestly thought this was the beginning of a miscarriage. That somehow my suppressed guilt over this pregnancy and stress caused this to happen. I called the doctor from the bathroom floor, wanting some answers and direction. Hope.

A short while later I found myself talking to a nurse who advised me to relax, and prop my feet up for the rest of the day. I was also due for another appointment in a few days, and things would either go very wrong, very quickly or get better. We both knew that nothing could be done at twelve weeks to save this baby. But being able to talk to someone and have them listen to my fears meant a lot. It wasn't even a lot of blood but it was enough to shake up our world that day.

To my utter amazement the spotting stopped, and I found myself sighing at my next appointment when little man's heartbeat was found, and all was well. But knowing that I could call any hour, of any day and have the support I needed was a blanket of comfort I needed so desperately. In addition to having strong emotional support from friends and family, it is just as important, if not more important to be surrounded by a medical staff during your pregnancy that will accommodate your inevitable anxiety over this new pregnancy. The things that were once 'little things' have a way of becoming monsters in subsequent pregnancy, and sometimes the only way to get peace of mind is hearing the baby's heart beat in between scheduled appointments, getting to talk to a nurse about your fears or seeing them swoosh around on the ultrasound monitor. My hope is that you have this medical and professional support - not just for your baby but for your well-being as well. I think it can be safe to say that in most cases - in pregnancy, and even in motherhood - taking care for yourself is taking care for your children.

Chapter 6

BONDING, THE BITTERSWEETNESS AND THE BIRTH

The moments following Joseph's birth are mostly a blur. I was told he had to go to the NICU as a precaution since he was born shortly before 36 weeks. My heart felt somewhat prepared for this. We had done this before. This time our baby had weeks and weeks of growth on his side. He was an incredible size - 7 pounds, 5 ounces - for a premature baby.

If you knew my doctor, you would know her first impression can be harsh. Over time you learn to love her because her devotion to the mother's and child's well-being are irrefutable. But the day she delivered Joseph I saw a different side of her. Maybe it's stories like this that make her job all worth it. I have often wondered how she does it. From the few years I have been going to her office, I've come to learn that they deal a lot with sad stories, broken hearts and crushed families. She saw our world ripped apart the day she had to confirm the bad news about our daughter's restricted growth. We second-guessed a lot of her findings, but ultimately came to love and trust her. Namely, we wanted to choose hope for as long as possible but from what she could see, week after week through the ultrasound appointments with Jenna, it was nearly impossible to render any scant of hope to us.

I knew that deep down inside everything was going to be alright. NICU or no NICU. He was born at 6:33 p.m. I saw our doctor beaming with pure happiness as she carried this beautiful new baby off to the nurses. Her grin went from ear to ear, as she realized this baby was bigger than even she anticipated.

I was able to hold him for a bit. *Hear his cry.*

Yes. This is how it was supposed to be.

I began to cry as he let out his first sound in this world. The nurse asked me if I was alright.

Oh yes, more than alright. Perfect, actually. I just nodded, and smiled through tears.

I didn't say anything. I only longed to hold him again. Hold my own child. The child I so longed for, so loved and so hoped for. The child that would restore so much hope and love into my heart and world.

I remember visiting him shortly after the c-section in the NICU, as they wheeled my entire bed over to where he was. The strangest feeling overcame me. This incredulous feeling of meeting someone for the first time, even though you've known them all along but still not recognizing them at first.

So this was the beautiful little boy who was growing inside me the entire time! The nights and early mornings of kicking, the hiccups... the life. Life would never, ever be the same.

Once again guilt brushed me, but only lightly. I felt like I was encompassed in this bubble again, but only this time to protect my heart from the relentless waves of grief. I knew that this joy of motherhood was something I deserved to be completely smothered in, and giving into it was in no way replacing my daughter, or forgetting our loss. This was a time of celebration, bittersweet tears, and even healing.

Our son was perfection. He laid there, asleep and completely unaware of the healing God was sending down through his little soul to ours.

He was a healthy, beautiful boy with big eyes, and soft, dark brown hair. He was a bit swollen, but I kept hearing that it was normal for c-section babies. I must have been there for some time, but it definitely did not feel long enough.

My nurses were pushing me to rest, and assured me that our son would be just fine.

Against my will, I was separated from my boy. My body needed the rest. I must have slept but still felt pretty tired even after the rest.

The next thing I can remember is being my postpartum room with my husband the next morning, impatiently waiting for a status report from a nurse. The bond was an incredible force already. I suppose it isn't shocking at all, seeing how he had been a part of me for almost nine months. I desperately missed my boy. We decided to take a chance and visit the NICU ourselves. I climbed into a wheelchair and we made it down there in a matter of minutes.

When we arrived we were told Joseph was being discharged out of the NICU. *It was like music to my ears!*

You go your entire life without ever knowing this little person, but the second you find out about them, meet them, hold them - you are never, ever the same and feel so incomplete without their presence. It is no wonder the *loss* of a child is just as devastating.

Over the next few days in the hospital for my postpartum stay, after the c-section, our room was constantly full of friends and family anxious to meet our little man and celebrate his life with us. He was a content little boy, sleeping quite a bit the first few days - during the day. I must have looked like a zombie those first few days - like I hadn't slept in weeks. I felt it too. None of it mattered though, I was smitten in the purest love over this amazing little boy. It didn't feel real that he was really *ours.*

I have to give God all the glory that grief did not rob me of joy those first few days. I suppose it might even have to do with the fact that my pregnancy with him wasn't all that smooth either, especially toward the end. I kept going into premature labor, and had multiple hospital stays toward the end. It felt like a huge sigh of relief to have him here, safe in my arms.

The 36 week mark we were originally aiming for his birth date, was about a week after the death date of my daughter. The entire thing was bittersweet, beyond words.

The more the contractions came, the more we all realized he would be coming sooner than we had hoped.

The dates were quickly starting to sound a lot like the dates surrounding our daughter's birth date. I begged our doctor to give this baby his own date. His own date for birthday cake, birthday balloons, birthday gifts, birthday celebrations. She granted our wish, and seemed to understand how important it would be to us not only now, but in the years ahead. She took him two days before Jenna's first birthday.

When her first birthday did finally roll around, Joseph had been discharged from the NICU, but since I had had a c-section I was still hospital bound. There is no easy way to say this - it just plain sucked.

That day *was* awful. That day was filled with all kinds of emotions. I mostly felt like a horrible mother to my daughter. Here I was, celebrating - when she was all alone, at the cemetery. My husband was able to visit her, but it still wasn't the same. I wanted to be there. I wanted the liberty to be nothing but devastated on her first birthday. I wanted to cry bitter tears over her headstone. That jarred feeling that grief often brings, settled over me that day. It was one of those emotions you try so hard to explain but end up more confused before just giving up. Never in a million years would I have chosen to leave the hospital to visit her graveside, but it still somehow felt wrong to not be there on such a significant day.

This was the first time I was introduced to the world of parenting after loss. I could no longer manage the things in my world around my grief, as before. This beautiful new boy of ours took precedence, even over my grief. And that - that awful reality that sometimes you just simply cannot grieve and be present for your living children at the same time - was all new to me. It stung in so many ways - for my son, and for my daughter. I was used to having the luxury, for lack of a better word, of visiting my daughter when I pleased, crying for her when I felt like I needed a good cry, powering up my laptop and writing when I felt the need to release pent up emotions.

It would be a long time, years even, before I could be gentle on myself for all the times that I couldn't be present in grief in this new world of mothering a child on earth.

Chapter 7

EMBRACING PARENTHOOD AND GRIEF

When we brought our son home to our small suburban house in Texas, you might have mistaken his room for a storage space. There was baby furniture we hadn't ever had the chance to use with his big sister, and there were boxes of diapers and other boxed up baby goods. The nursery was anything but ready for him. It looked and felt like an abandoned baby room. And that is exactly what it was, at least until he was born.

These are mistakes I made with him, the mistakes I am trying desperately to do differently with our last child. And maybe, in retrospect they weren't mistakes at all. I was surviving and doing everything I possibly could. It was all I could do to get the things we needed, tuck them away in his own room, and not mess with them until absolutely necessary - which would essentially be him, here, with us. But it rings in my heart like a regret. I did not spend a whole lot of time planning for his arrival, save the essentials for bringing home a baby like the carseat, the monitor and the breast pump. Looking back, I wish I would have spent time decorating his room. Making it cozy and perfect. Spending some time, carrying his growing self inside me, in his room where so much of his life would be spent. Preparing his nursery before he was born felt like I could be jinxing our future, and setting ourselves up for more disappointment. It also felt like replacement. This furniture should have been more worn, and broken in by a big sister. It was brand new and yet it had been purchased and sitting in our presence for over a year.

Mothering our son during the first few weeks was a sacred time. I was in constant awe over his littleness, his perfection, his big eyes and olive skin. Everything about this little person fascinated me, from his sleeping little body to his facial expressions, to watching him as he discovered the world around him. Watching his little chest rise and fall as he slept was indescribable. I spent so much time those first few months wonderstruck over how *life* came so easy to this little man of ours. The fact that he could breathe without any medical support, to me, was a miracle I could barely get over. And then to top it all off was the growing faith that he would be ours to stay. Motherhood is a privilege beyond words, something that could only be thought up by such an amazing Creator.

A few weeks after he was born we found ourselves wanting to take family pictures for the first time. I was caught off guard by grief in the sense that it just felt so incomplete without our daughter. I remember grasping for ideas through the blogs I followed, trying to see how others included their children in Heaven in their family portraits. Ultimately I decided to wear a piece of jewelry that I remembered her by, not the most creative way to include our daughter but I loved the subtle addition. It somehow made the photo session more complete.

For a little while after our son was born, a cloud of darkness fell over me. It was something that did not last long, but was profound in the way it tormented me. Looking at this amazing little boy, day after day, moment by moment was becoming a constant reminder of all the beautiful things I missed out on with our daughter. Bitter tears fell every time I thought about how I never got to rock her, sing to her, read to her or watch her sleep so peacefully in our living room.

When grief would overwhelm me, I would find myself cuddling this beautiful boy of mine close, letting the tears fall over his soft head. I felt like a horrible mother. The world around me, my own heart even, was begging me to be okay, but inside I still longed for these moments with her.

Over the span of a few weeks since his birth, his looks were changing almost daily. One thing that remained the same though was his silhouette. His silhouette reminded me so much of the 'Cox nose' that our daughter inherited from her Daddy. I was thankful to Heaven for the resemblance. It was a glimpse of her in him. A piece of her that lived on, a beautiful family resemblance that both my children shared. Little things like this helped that cloud of darkness disappear over time, and enjoy what was right before my eyes. A precious son, but also a glimpse. A much needed, much craved glimpse of what she might have been like.

One of the most disturbing things about parenting after loss is living with the fear that you have somehow let down your living children. Filling out paperwork has a way of messing with your head. In such a seemingly meaningless way too. When the forms at the doctors' offices ask for siblings, I can't help but wonder... why. On Joseph's pediatric forms at his first check up after birth, there was even a place on the form that asked if any siblings had passed away, and how. Obviously there must be a reason, but filling in that information on the form made the guilt rise to the surface.

Have I damaged my son somehow? Did it mean that I was less of a mother because I could say 'yes, I have a child that did not survive'. Would the doctors and nurses see my answer and question my ability as a mother?

He must have been only a few weeks old when I told my husband I really needed a visit to the cemetery. I missed out on going on her first birthday, her death date, and as more time slipped by, the more guilt I felt in not being able to go.

We drove together one afternoon, and Joseph was fast asleep in the carseat. We lugged him over to her spot in the ground, rested his carseat on the grass and sat in silence. I wondered how he would be affected by this over time. Having a dead sister. I pitied him, that he didn't have a say in the matter - being brought into a home where so much loss had taken place. As a mother I longed to protect him.

But inside a window of light was begging for more of my attention. We went to the cemetery quite a bit for the first two years, and we always brought him with us. I began to realize that growing up so close to death, might make him more sensitive, more compassionate, and maybe even more aware of Heaven. That would be my honest hope anyway. He most definitely did not have a say in the way he was brought into the world, but he could be incredible because of it. I decided it was good to bring him to the cemetery. Being so close to death might make life more precious for him over the years.

As this new normal was settling so comfortably into our lives, there was something I yearned for still. The new normal was even more incredible than I thought it could be. More okay than I ever hoped for. And just like grief, the problem came from life carrying on, passing through as if nothing had ever happened. It might sound crazy but the raw grief that feels like your chest is being ripped open - that intense sadness that you think will never leave your heart - it made me feel close to my daughter. Close to her tiny existence. Close to her being real. Close to everything that had to do with her. The moments of intense sadness were becoming further and further apart. While it was refreshing to be able to enjoy things in life again, without so much grief and guilt weighing on my mind, it was also a strange place to find myself. Strange that as a mother, I could be okay with one of my children gone. I actually missed the raw moments of grief. When a good cry would overcome me, I would soon find myself interrupted with the needs of my beautiful son. It wasn't all about me and my grief anymore, but I did long for a time that I could be in that moment, for as long as needed, to feel close to the child that left our world much too soon.

It became increasingly obvious, with the demands of an infant, that I would not have the time to grieve freely, but I could make the time. Making time for just my daughter was important for so many reasons. It helped me focus more on my son while he was awake, and it made it okay that I could not grieve as I used to. The best time for me was usually in the evening, after my son and husband had turned in for the night. I would make time for her through reading books and blogs, creating cards for the bereaved community, and connecting with loss moms. Sometimes it even helped to get out her things, and spend some time looking through the scrapbook of her NICU stay I put together for her funeral.

Your schedule might look a lot different, but it can be helpful to find a time during your day, or even week for your child gone too soon. I found that when I was unable to make time just for her, I was not functioning like I should. I needed that time with her, as much as I needed it with my husband and son.

Chapter 8

CELEBRATING YOUR NEW BABY NOW:
BEFORE THEY ARRIVE

It wasn't until we fell pregnant with our last child, the one I am currently carrying at the time of writing this book, that I realized I remember so little about my pregnancy with our son - our first rainbow baby. I remember so much from my very first pregnancy, the one with Jenna. Back when pregnancy was simple. Before the innocence was gone.

Of course the timing of the beginning of my pregnancy with him was well within the first year of heavy grief too. Everything seems foggy that first year. But that realization that I can remember so few details, when really it should be the one I can remember the most, was incredibly sad to me. I didn't know any better than to just get through it. Survive. What I do remember is loving being pregnant. Looking back, I only wish I had made more effort to journal, take pictures - do something to make memories those beautiful months my boy was growing inside me.

However, if surviving is all you can do, you've done more than enough. But my hope in writing this book is to help you make memories... now. Celebrate your beautiful new baby... now. You deserve happiness in pregnancy again, and even when it is hard to come by - you are not alone - no matter what you might be feeling.

Since becoming pregnant with what most likely be our last child, it is a bittersweet end to be experiencing all the big and little things about pregnancy. I feel passionately about making this a memorable time with her. I piled a list that I hope inspires you to capture this time in your life with your baby as well.

First Trimester

Make a list of names for your baby. Have fun with this. You might already be doing this, and then again you might be holding off until you hear a heartbeat for the first time. Whichever choice you make will be the right one for you, but don't be afraid to let yourself dream of your little one and what you hope to name them. Name choosing is one of the best things you get to do while pregnant.

Start a journal. You might be sick all day, everyday, and then again you might be one of the lucky ones who don't ever experience much, if any, morning sickness. If you find yourself too drained or unmotivated to write down tidbits from your pregnancy journey, try to make a time - even if it's just once a week - to reflect on how things are coming along with you and the baby. Right now it might seem minuscule, but one day it will be a journal you will treasure. Don't underestimate the power and incredulous journey you are on. Your words will empower you in the days ahead, and show you how far you've come.

Create your mantra and write it on an index card. Place it somewhere you can see it daily. Your mantra might be a verse you've claimed for this pregnancy, it might be a quote, or it might be a few words that empower you each day to keep your head up high when all you can think of is feeling guilty or fear.

Start a Prayer Journal. Yes, another writing assignment, but this one is a little different. Write down your prayers, and date them. Maybe start by praying something small, like praying you will make it to the next week without any complications. When that prayer has been answered, highlight it. The more prayers you record, and see answered, the more your hope and faith may increase, which is only beneficial for your baby.

Take a picture of your bump. It might not be very noticeable yet, but it will be neat to keep track of your growing belly through weekly or even monthly snapshots.

Start a charm bracelet, or if you have one - add a charm that represents this new pregnancy. You can add to the bracelet throughout the years.

Tell others the news. You might even find a fun and unique way to share, such as wrapping up "I love my Grandma" onesies, or make copies of your ultrasound picture and placing it in a picture frame.

SECOND TRIMESTER

Consider gifting yourself with a Mexican Bola Necklace.
The Mexican Bola Necklace is a beautiful way to begin the bonding process as your baby's hearing develops in the second trimester. As the baby's hearing improves she may come to familiarize the soft chime of the Bola Necklace with comfort, even well after birth.

Read your favorite children's book to your baby. One of my personal favorites is the book "Wherever You Are" by Nancy Tillman. While you might be tempted to distance yourself as much as possible from this new pregnancy, for fear of losing the baby, be gentle on yourself. Those feelings are normal, and nothing to be ashamed about. It is only natural to want to protect your heart from even more heartbreak and disappointment. Make a little time to begin the bonding process. Reading to your baby can help you form this bond early. When I read this book, I always feel like I am reading to all my babies - even the one I can't hold on this earth anymore. That is comforting somehow.

Start a scrapbook. By now you have most likely collected a handful of ultrasound pictures, maybe a few appointment cards and other mementos from this pregnancy. You can start by laying out the first few pages and decorating. If this is overwhelming you can take it slow and spend 10-15 minutes at a time laying out your pictures and mementos to get ideas.

Relax with some music. Play it for yourself, and the baby in the days that are the most difficult. Turn off the television, close your laptop, turn off your phone, let all the distractions take the back plate for just a bit. Let your mind rest, and listen the words or the rhythm of the song. You might even take this opportunity to light a candle of your favorite scent. In the years to come when you hear the music, it will remind you of this bittersweet journey and how far you've come.

Find a good book that has nothing to do with pregnancy, newborns or babies. It's all about distractions right now, so if you're into romance novels, finding new recipes, reading up on the latest celebrity gossip - try to make sure they are within your grasp.

Start a Pinterest Dream Board. This may not be something you are comfortable doing, but I found great freedom in allowing myself to embrace new ideas for a nursery, wall decorations and more for our newest little one. Somehow it was even sweeter than I imagined it to be, and not nearly as scary. Visit Pinterest.com if you do not already have an account and you can begin by creating a board for your beautiful new baby. The best part about this is, you can even make the board private, in case sharing this with the outside world is too much.

Talk to your baby. This might sound redundant, and something you hear in all the baby books, but in a subsequent pregnancy after loss, bonding can be an upward battle in so many ways. Don't be afraid to talk to your sweet baby growing inside. It is very likely they can hear you somewhere around 20 weeks.

THIRD TRIMESTER

Register. The weeks might feel like years, but your baby's arrival is closer than it might feel. Be sure to use this time to register for all the baby things you need *and* want. It is extremely likely that people in your world not only want to buy you things for this new baby -- they want to celebrate this new miracle with you by giving a little extra. While they most likely do not understand the extent of your pain nor your journey, many of them are aware that this hasn't been a cake walk for you either. Let them spoil you with gifts, and enjoy filling up that registry. You deserve this moment, and you deserve the right to dream for your future.

Baby Shower. We talked about this a little in the last chapter, but if you are one of those rock stars I was talking about, I say go for it! Let your beautiful friends and family shower you with presents, hugs, well wishes, cards -- even tears of joy for a few hours. And who doesn't love cake? There is no doubt it will be bittersweet, even if only on the inside, but it is a huge step in healing and embracing this new life and new normal.

Write your birth plan. You might be, and then again you might not be that mother who has her well written birth plan ready weeks in advance, but writing a birth plan can not only be helpful for you and those who will be near you when the baby makes his or her arrival, but it can be an exciting time to reflect on the joy that awaits.

Treat yourself to a prenatal massage and pedicure. As with anything else, you should consult with your doctor before scheduling a prenatal massage, but massage therapy during pregnancy has been proven to be extremely beneficial for expecting mothers well into their third trimesters - including hormone regulation, help in reduction of edema, reduced stress and much more.

Start a Prayer Quilt. It's time to break out that prayer journal. If you don't know how to quilt, find a friend that does, or even find a good tutorial on YouTube to make a simple one. Really, all you need right now are fabric squares. The actual quilt can be sewn together by someone who knows how to quilt, if you are unable to at a later date. Grab a stack full of quilt blocks, and begin writing all the prayers that have been answered over the past few months. Date each square if you have the dates available. You could even mix in some verses on some squares, or quotes or song lyrics that you enjoy. Enjoy gathering the colors and patterned fabrics for the quilt.

Schedule maternity photos. It seems like all the big stuff (and the FUN stuff) is this trimester! Enjoy it, mama. You deserve it. I can't say that enough. You might have a friend that is willing to document this beautiful, growing belly of yours, or you might want to scope out a photographer in your area. Either way, be sure to celebrate this last stretch of pregnancy with pictures that you will treasure in the years to come.

Celebrate your growing belly with some belly art. You can have someone paint a beautiful design on your belly, have a reputable artist apply some henna art, or even have a belly cast done. Be sure to document your belly art with tons of pictures! (be sure to consult your doctor ahead of time on these to ensure safety)

Consider having a Blessingway in addition to or instead of a baby shower. Traditionally a baby shower is focused on the arrival of the baby (and rightfully so) but a Blessingway, also known as a Mother Blessing, is intended to foster to the needs of the mother, and help her work through any issues she might be dealing with internally. The Blessingway is intended only for close friends and family of the mother, and usually only for women. You might pick up the book "Mother Rising" for in depth details on how to plan for a Blessingway.

Conclusion

Don't be afraid to listen to your instincts, and lean on grief even after bringing a new child into this world. As just about any rainbow mama can tell you, bringing new life into this world heals huge parts of your world and heart, but grief will continue her work in you forever. She is a permanent part of your life. It is imperative to your continual healing to make time for that sacred expression of love - as much or as little as that may be.

It is my earnest hope that you might carry this new baby with a sense of revived joy, and courage. Pregnancy after loss is a terrifying time that few can truly understand. Think of this incredible journey as a challenge. A challenge to not only enjoy this beautiful gift you have been chosen to bear, but write history by cherishing and documenting this time in your life. Dare to unravel the ferocious grips of grief and guilt over your heart. You, more than most, deserve this.

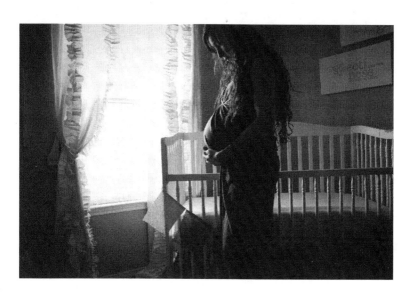

Sending a heartfelt thanks for allowing me
the space and opportunity to share our story of hope,
loss and love with you. May your journey
be filled with more hope and healing
than you ever dreamed possible.

Made in the USA
Middletown, DE
10 October 2016